Disclaimer

This book is intended as a reference material, not as a medical manual to replace the advice of your physician or to substitute for any treatment prescribed by your physician.

If you are ill or suspect that you have a medical problem, we strongly encourage you to consult your medical, health, or other competent professional before adopting any of the suggestions in this book or drawing inferences from it. If you are taking prescription medication, you should never change your diet (for better or worse) without consulting your physician, as any dietary change may affect the metabolism of that prescription drug.

This book and the author's opinions are solely for informational and educational purposes.

The author specifically disclaims all responsibility for any liability, loss, or risk, personal or otherwise which is incurred as a consequence, directly or indirectly, of the use and application of any of the contents of this book. Individual results may vary.

Published by:

Nick Stanton and Random Technologies

4409 HOFFNER AVENUE, SUITE 347

Belle Isle, FL 32812

Website: http://www.Lose15in5Days.com

E-Mail: support@Lose15in5Days.com

Table of Contents

<u>Introduction</u>

I know what you're thinking. You have tried numerous diets, failed to lose weight in the past and you are wondering how this diet plan will be any different. Here is my answer. Many diet plans offer what I like to call lose-weight quick schemes. What do I mean by that? Many diet plans help you lose the weight for only a short time, but offers no long term-plan to keep the weight off. To keep the weight at bay in other diet plans you would have to deprive yourself of certain foods for life. That's no way to live.

Unlike other diets which restrict certain foods and deprive you of vital nutrients, my diet plan does not require you to give up any kind of food while eating smaller portions, getting vital nutrients and exercising regularly.

That's it. No complicated scientific methods, no health nuts looking over your shoulder. This plan is about you getting to know your body and eating the foods you love while eating new foods which are beneficial to your health.

Thank You For Your Investment

This diet plan is probably unlike any other diet plan you have tried in the past. Not only will this diet work, but it will keep the weight off and keep you at your desired weight. This is not a typical fad diet; it is a long-term diet plan which finally sheds those unwanted pounds.

I am not a doctor or any form of health professional. I am an average person and I know that the daily routine of work, stress and carting the kids to school can hinder us from eating the right foods and setting a solid, exercise routine. Therefore, I have created a diet plan that will integrate successfully with your busy schedule.

<u>This is not just simply a diet, but a new way of living.</u>

Bottom line, the key to this diet is not a complex, scientific diet, but a simple common sense approach to dieting and exercise.

The keyword is COMMON SENSE because this diet is focused on sensible eating and exercise.

You may already know some of the information in this plan and I will provide you more tools to better help you manage your weight.

This is a diet plan that works and has consistently worked for me to this day.

How Lose 15 In 5 Works

The diet plan is a simple, easy-to-follow method to lose your desired weight.

Follow this diet for five days at a time. Repeat as necessary for more stubborn weight loss, or until you reach the desired weight you have in mind.

This program can be repeated 2 times in a row, but break for 1-2 weeks. When your break is over, continue the plan as normal.

Not eating for 5 days will not get you to your desired weight. Eat, drink and prepare as necessary.

All preparation foods can be found at your local grocery store.

Important Key Points:

Before You Begin

1. All prepared foods should either be <u>boiled, steamed, broiled or grilled.</u>
2. No oils, salts, bread, potatoes, rice, starch alcohol etc.

3. Use only white vinegar, lemon juice, lime juice, chili pepper, black pepper and dried herbs to season food.
4. Eat only fresh foods prepared by you alone. Do not eat canned or prepared foods. They contain salts, oils, fats, sugar and other additives.
5. If you do not eat red meat, you can substitute with 3oz. tuna (in water), salmon (4 - 6oz.) or skinless chicken breast chicken (4 – 6oz.) or half a cup of firm tofu.
6. NO SNACKING.

7. No strenuous exercising during the 5 day diet phase, but exercise before or after is fine. You may ask yourself why. Statistically, those who have tried the plan attain better results when they DO NOT exercise excessively.

8. Drink at least 7 - 12 cups (250 ml/8 fl. oz.) of water per day, 2 cups of water when waking up, 2 cups of water before bed and 1 cup of water before each meal.

Lose The Weight And Keep It Off

Here are a few simple points when starting the plan.

Do not waste your money by throwing away old food in your refrigerator or kitchen cabinets. Instead, understand proportions and calories. Read the back of food labels and learn to place your favorite meals in proper proportion. With this diet plan, there are no sudden changes so do not do yourself the disservice of abruptly changing what you eat.

Eat whatever you want. Do not deny yourself any kind of food, even the unhealthy ones. Denying yourself certain foods will cause massive cravings and eventual overeating of those foods you tried to resist. Instead, eat the unhealthy foods you crave in smaller portions. Read food labels and understand calories and servings charts.

i.e. 1 cup water = 0 cal vs. 1 cup cola = 160 calories, 13 tsp. sugar

For example: My children and I love to eat at our local hamburger restaurant so instead of having a soda with my meal I will have water. I eat un-salted regular fries, baked potato or salad, and I order a single patty burger instead of a double or triple with no mayonnaise or cheese. Not only did I make the right choices and not deny myself the favorite foods I crave, but I also set an excellent example for my children; they now drink water instead of soda with their meals.

While you can still enjoy your favorite foods, condition your body to accept different types of foods, especially foods that are rich in nutrients and vitamins. Because your body feeds off those nutrients, you will naturally gravitate towards those healthy foods just as your favorite unhealthy foods.

Health Tip: Foods that are rich in nutrients satisfy cravings better than junk food.

Satisfy your hunger, not your desires.

Do not eat when starving. Eat when you're hungry. Eating when starving will cause overeating. To remedy this, eat healthy snacks between major meals.

Healthy Snacks

5 carrot or celery sticks with half a teaspoon of hummus on each stick. Choose hummus that contains no salt, made from olive oil (no other oils like canola or soy) and preferably organic. A few dashes of hot sauce can be added if you like your snacks spicy.

A small handful of raw (not roasted) unsalted nuts. Choose from any of your favorite - almonds, cashews, peanuts, walnuts etc.

3 celery sticks with half a teaspoon of peanut butter on each stick.
Any combination of 10 raw vegetable sticks - carrot, peppers, cucumber, celery, snap peas for dipping into fresh salsa. Do not use salsa from a jar as it's processed. Either buy the fresh salsa in the cold deli

section of the supermarket (read the label to make sure its vegetables and natural herbs and spices only) or make your own by mixing chopped tomatoes, onions, cilantro and jalapenos with a squeeze of lime juice.

Craving something sweet? Try:
A half-inch thick slice of watermelon
10 frozen grapes

*Limit to 2 healthy snacks a day

Get to know your body by knowing how many calories to consume per day. Quite simply, IF THE AMOUNT EXCEEDS YOUR BODY'S CALORIE INTAKE THEN YOU WILL GAIN WEIGHT.
Health Fact: In Italy, Italians eat larger meals at lunch time while eating lighter

meals during the day. Where am I going with this?

Eating heavier calories during breakfast and lunch will allow you to burn more calories during the day while reserving the least amount of calories for when you are not as active towards the late afternoon and evening.

Get up from the table and leave after eating your meal. It takes around 20 minutes for the brain to let your body know that you are full. It may seem awkward and jarring at first, but let others know what you are doing and as you practice it will become natural. If after 20 minutes you are still hungry, and by hungry I mean that your body craves more calories, then sit back down and continue eating. DO NOT overfill yourself.

Short-term effects of overeating: lack of energy, feeling bloated, tiredness and possible queasiness.

Long-term effects of overeating: weight-gain, no longer fitting into clothes, unhappiness with weight, more overeating and health risks.

REMEMBER: It takes around 20-30 minutes to eat and 2-4 hours to fully digest food.

You may ask yourself why you overeat over and over again and here is why. You are not reminded of the short and long term effects of overeating. If you know the consequences of overeating while eating your meals, your willpower will kick in and you WILL NOT overeat. If necessary, place a list of the short and long-term effects of overeating near your dining area.

REMEMBER: We're all human and there are times when you will overeat. Do not worry. It happens to me as well. . . Just get back on the saddle and keeping following the diet plan. YOU CAN AND WILL LOSE THE WEIGHT!

AND FINALLY: Exercise.

That's right; I said it. Exercise is ESSENTIAL to good health. But don't overdo it while on the program, at least 30 minutes of activity 3 to 4 times per week will dramatically contribute to your overall weight loss and fitness.

If you follow these simple steps and get to know your body you will lose the weight.

Losing those unwanted pounds will improve your physical, mental and emotional health.

Building Healthy Eating Habits

Most people fail and don't stick to their 'diets' as it just becomes all too hard with everyday life. Things such as working too late, no motivation to cook after a long day, unexpected events and emergencies makes it very easy just to take the easy path of the fast food drive-thru for something quick.

Also many people resent 'diets' as they feel deprived and/or hungry and even events like going out to a restaurant with family or friends can become stressful. In the end it all just becomes too hard.

Here are a few helpful tips that will keep you on track and build better eating habits while on The Lose 15 In 5 Days™ System or not.

<u>Grocery Shopping</u>

Prepare a full shopping list for your 5 days of everything you need and stick to it. Don't purchase anything else.

Go to the supermarket once only for the week and purchase everything you need for the 5 days. That way you have everything on hand and it's done. You have your eating plan and now you don't have to think about it.

When you are not on The Lose 15 In 5 Days™ System get into the habit of planning your meals for the week and creating your shopping list. If you have a shopping list, you will be more focused and less likely to stray to unhealthy things. It takes a few minutes, but saves time in running back to the store for missed ingredients.

The first few visits, give yourself enough time to shop. Be sure to take your time, as you should check the labels of ingredients. Once mastered, it won't take as long as you will know what items to purchase and what to avoid.

Avoid shopping when hungry. This will lead to over-purchases and temptations to buy other unnecessary items.

Shop on product delivery days if possible; ask your grocer when the store receives fresh produce. Fruits and veggies lose nutrients and flavor the longer they sit out in the air and light.

Purchase fruits at every trip to the grocery store and keep a supply on hand to provide healthy, filling snacks and can be used to satisfy your sweet tooth. Buy a wide variety of fruits to add flavor and boost the nutrition levels of your snacks. Some healthy fruit choices include: oranges, apples, kiwi, grapefruit, watermelon, honeydew, cantaloupe, grapes and tangerines.

Try not to shop with your kids or spouse. You know they will want those sweets and chips.

<u>Eating Out</u>

If you have to eat out while on The Lose 15 In 5 Days™ System tell the waiter exactly what you want even if it is not on the menu.

State you want a grilled skinless chicken breast with a side of steamed zucchini or mixed vegetables. Most restaurants want to please your taste buds not your waist line and that is why you won't find this on a menu. Many restaurants will accommodate to your dietary needs, so you'll leave a happy customer and likely return.

Many restaurants now have their menus online, if you want to dine out and you are on your off week then look up their menu and plan what you are going to order. This gives you plenty of time to look over the choices and chose something healthy instead of being tempted and ordering something on impulse.

As soon as the bread basket hits the table tell the waiter you don't want it and to take it away or tell them not to bring it at all when being seated. Little things like this won't tempt you to overeat, and if it's not there you won' feel deprived.

Eat a small healthy snack before leaving for the restaurant. Never arrive at a restaurant hungry. Hungry people make bad ordering decisions and you won't be tempted buy that cheeseburger and fries.

Eat slowly and savor each bit. Enjoy the conversation at the table. Put your knife and fork down between bites. Don't pick it up again until you've completely swallowed the last bite. Provide your body time to digest.

Be the first to order at the table. This way you won't be tempted by what others order.

Start with a salad. Filling your empty stomach with a salad before a meal is a good way to keep you from binging on your entrée later. Be selective. A garden salad will help hold you over until your entrée arrives. When you order a salad, go for the olive oil and vinegar dressing and ask for it on the side so you can control how much you use. Try dipping your fork lightly in the dressing to eat with each bite. This way, you have control over how much or how little you add. Beware of salads like chicken Caesar salad, as it is often higher in fat and calories than a cheeseburger.

Portion sizes in restaurants can be more than you need. If you receive too large a portion, eat only half. When you feel full, stop eating. You do not need to finish your meal. Just because it's there doesn't mean you have to eat it! Ask for a takeout box or doggy bag, and take it home for another meal. Keep your portions under control when you are dining out. Try to never eat until full, but only satisfied.

Drink water. A good way to avoid sugar filled drinks is to get water and/or unsweetened tea. Drink a lot of water before your meals to make you fuller and less likely to overeat.

Alcohol can stimulate your appetite which leads to overeating and drinking loosens your inhibitions and may make you eat without thinking. Plus the calories in alcohol can add up fast. If you must have an alcoholic drink then order a glass of wine and sip slowly on it through your dinner. Drink lots of water as your eat to quench your thirst and help you nurse your alcohol drink.

If it's a special occasion and you must have a dessert then share it with one of your companions. Opt for a healthier alternative like sorbet or fresh fruit.

Avoid buffets. Portion control can become a foreign concept for almost everybody at an all-you-can-eat buffet. The sheer variety of foods available at buffets is also daunting. Studies have shown that when we're given more choices, we tend to eat more without realizing it. Simply avoid buffet restaurants and you won't have to face this temptation.

<u>General</u>

Stay asleep longer. Getting to bed just 30 minutes earlier and waking up 30 minutes later than you normally do can help you make better food choices. Also, when you're well-rested, you're less prone to snacking out of fatigue or stress.

When you are not on The Lose 15 In 5 Days™ System start slow and make changes to your eating habits over time. Trying to make your diet healthy overnight isn't realistic or smart. Changing everything at once usually leads to cheating or giving up on your new eating plan. Make small steps, like adding a salad (full of different colored vegetables) to your diet once a day or switching from butter to olive oil or to steaming when cooking. As your small changes become habit, you can continue to add more healthy choices to your diet.

Every change you make to improve your diet matters. You don't have to be perfect and you don't have to completely eliminate foods you enjoy to have a healthy diet. The long term goal is to feel good, have more energy, and be healthier.

Overindulged? It happens. Christmas, Thanksgiving, office parties. Don't let your missteps derail you or make you want to give up. Expect setbacks. Everyone is bound to give in to temptation from time to time. The danger isn't a single splurge but letting it become an excuse for an all-out binge. Call it the "I've already blown it so I might as well eat the entire bag of cookies" syndrome.

Try not to think of certain foods as "off-limits." When you ban certain foods or food groups, it is natural to want those foods more, and then feel like a failure if you give in to temptation. If you are drawn towards sweet, salty, or unhealthy foods, start by reducing portion sizes and not eating them as often. Later you may find yourself craving them less or thinking of them as only occasional indulgences.

Tell people you're on a new eating plan. There is no reason to be ashamed that you want to lose weight and be healthier. In fact, telling your coworkers, family etc. will increase your accountability. It will motivate you that they know because you will not want to fail. Some of them may become your greatest motivators.

Reward Yourself. A new healthier way of living can be hard work at first. Small rewards can provide an incentive to keep going. But make sure your rewards are not food-related. (Translation: Rewarding yourself for losing 5 pounds with a box of chocolates is not what we're talking about.) Set mini-goals along the way and reward yourself when you reach them. Your reward could be a massage, a new haircut or style, a movie or a new pair of jeans. Celebrating your success will keep you on track and your resolve to continue.

Answers To Common Questions

a) **Question** – I'm uncertain what a 1 cup or ½ cup measurement is?

Answer - 1 cup is measured in volume not weight and is equal to 8 fluid ounces or 250ml i.e. ½ cup green beans is equal to 4 fluid ounces or 125ml.

b) **Question**- I'm uncertain about stewed tomatoes. How do I make stewed tomatoes?

Answer -The simplest way is to chop your tomatoes into 4 parts and cook them in a sauce pan or pot at medium heat for approximately 20-25 min.

c) **Question** – What is a hamburger patty?

Answer – A hamburger patty is also known as a beef burger which is ground beef only (lean if possible) that is formed into a puck shape

d) **Question** – I can't find certain fruits and vegetable because they are out of season.
Answer - If you cannot find particular fresh foods then you may use frozen (not canned) as long as they have not added any salt or sugar and preferably organic.

e) **Question** – When should I see the weight loss while on the 5 day plan?
Answer - The rate of weight loss varies for everyone, its best to check your weight on the morning after the 5th day.

f) **Question** – I don't drink coffee or tea, can I have herbal tea?

Answer - For best results drink regular (caffeinated) coffee or tea. But if it's impossible then drink herbal.

g) **Question**- I take vitamins & supplements, can I continue taking them?
Answer - Yes you may, vitamins are OK and supplements are as well long as they are not meal replacements.

h) **Question** – Can I buy my tomato juice?
Answer - Yes you may, but if possible try to buy low sodium tomato juice and read the label for any hidden sugars or additives.

i) **Question** Can I switch my meals around?
Answer - No, for best results follow the plan as prescribed.

j) **Question** -Can stay on the plan longer than 5 days?

Answer - Yes you can, you can repeat the plan once a week until you have reached your weight loss goal.

Thank you for choosing my Lose 15 in 5 Days program.

To gain access to printable versions of the shopping list and weekly food menu chart, that you can keep in your kitchen, on the refrigerator and reference when you go to the grocery store, please visit the following website:

www.subscribe.lose15in5days.com